The Complete Intermittent Fasting For Women Over 50

A Superlative Guide To Understanding The Concepts Of Intermittent Fasting Diet For Seniors; Master The Basics And Promote Health And Weight Loss Through Autophagy.

Anna Evans

Table Of Contents

INTRODUCTION

You may have heard about Intermittent Fasting from your friends, or maybe some random talk show mentioned it as some fat loss miracle. You've overheard some women at the gym bringing it up during their chat about carb-cycling and protein shakes, but what is it? The name says it all. Intermittent-periods; fasting—being without food. What's so special about periods without food? Every time I say the word fasting to my relatives, they get this big fearful look on their faces as if I am starving myself and could die at any moment! Fortunately, you won't be starving yourself. It's not one of those fasts that last 30 days and have you drinking lemonade and spices.

CHAPTER 1. HISTORY OF INTERMITTENT FASTING

When you feel the need to lose weight and cutting down your calories, you will find intermittent fasting the best way for sure. There are many ways by which you can reduce weight, but intermittent fasting or periodic fasting has many benefits apart from weight loss. Eating healthy, cutting down calories that are eating in a caloric deficit, and doing workouts will reduce weight. Here comes the question of how the idea of intermittent fasting came into being and who discovered it?

Fasting is an ancient ritual, which has been followed over the centuries by many cultures and religions. It is important to understand that fasting and starvation are two different things and shouldn't be mixed up. Starvation is a term used when the person has no idea about the availability of the meal, and there is a shortage of resources while fasting is avoiding the meals intentionally and the food is available.

Periodic fasting was used not just to cure the illnesses in ancient Egypt and Greece but also to prevent many diseases. Intermittent fasting was highly common in the middle Ages as people sought to enjoy its benefits. It was seen that intermittent fasting not only helps in reducing weight but also decreases insulin resistance. It is also used for the prevention of many diseases.

Intermittent fasting is the most common debate these days, so scientists are busy collecting intermittent fasting data. Studies conducted by Harvard have stated that fasting improves health, and those who practice intermittent fasting there are chances of increased life expectancy. This is quite obvious healthy individuals will survive longer because they will be physically active, and their body will be in the best state of health.

Intermittent fasting is both physical and religiously related. Many people practice intermittent fasting as part of their religion. Like Muslims, they fast in the holy month of Ramadan; Hindus observe different types of fasting according to their religion. Judaism has several common behaviors that include Yom Kippur, the truth of some. During the political times by a very famous leader Mahatma Gandhi at India's time of independence, Fasting was also observed.

In addition to controlling blood sugar, eating just one meal a day brings more benefits: reducing waist size and increasing muscle through the hormone HGH. Assuming the individual does not ingest non-protein foods, lowering blood pressure, improving lipid profile through lower LDL and higher HDL, reduced CRP or inflation, sound, even earlier, more significant over time as in any case, etc.

The concept of intermittent fasting has evolved with time. Starting from the point where it was considered starvation or due to insufficient sources, people used to stay hungry for a more extended period, the term fasting was identified. The definition of intermittent fasting has been changed from a period of fasting for hours or eating only one meal.

What Is Intermittent Fasting?

Intermittent fasting is described as an eating method that hovers between eating and fasting on a planned schedule. Several researchers have shown that this fasting method is very efficient for weight control and control of various kinds of diseases.

While several other diets focus on what you should eat, intermittent fasting focuses on what time to eat. Intermittent fasting restricts your eating plan to a specified period of the day, which, when followed, will make you lose weight, burn belly fat, and live a healthy life. There are several ways of doing intermittent fasting; yours is to study yourself and see the one that aligns with your health status and works best for you, then keep to it.

How Does Intermittent Fasting Work?

Even though there are several intermittent methods, the main routine of practicing all of them is to choose a pre-arranged period when you will eat and fast daily. An example is eating for 8 hours a day and fast for 16 hours, and you can also eat for five days of the weak and fast for the other two days (although both fasting days must not follow each other).

Intermittent fasting is different from the usual eating method because by eating three times a day together with snacks and not engaging in exercise, then you are only building your calories every time and not burning the fats storing in your body.

CHAPTER 2. BENEFITS OF INTERMITTENT FASTING FOR WOMEN OVER AGE 50

There are numerous benefits intermittent fasting has on the body of all humans and across all age groups. But in the course of this study, we are restricting our scope to women over 50. Some of these benefits are as follows:

<u>Reduction in the Risk of Cancer</u>

Intermittent fasting, which could also be referred to as mild caloric restriction, is very effective in the slowing down of fast-growing tumors that could lead to cancer.

Rous and Moreschi first discovered this benefit, and since then, it has gained wide recognition in the medical society. Restricting one's calorie intake also helps to boost the sensitivity of cancerous tumors to irradiation and chemotherapy.

Another benefit of intermittent fasting on women over 50 is the impairment of cancerous cells' metabolic process. This would make less energy available in the cell to function and most likely harm other cells.

Aside from that benefit, it serves to slow down, and if possible, shut down tumors, and it could help weaken them before treatments.

There is an action on transcription that boosts the effects of intermittent fasting against cancer. So, what is transcription? This is the process of copying information located in strands of DNA into molecular messengers called RNA.

The process is made possible by an enzyme known as RNA polymerase and many accessories of protein, which are classified as transcription factors. Some of these proteins include the forkhead box transcription factor (FOXO).

All the proteins play key roles in the process of metabolism, stress resistance, apoptosis (the programming process of cell death) as well as cellular proliferation (the process of cell growth).

Therefore, when this FOXO is activated during intermittent fasting, we could expect to see increased protection against carcinogenesis or tumorigenesis (the formation of cancer) and even the death of cancerous cells.

Another effect of FOXO's activation is increasing normal cells' resistance ability against stress, which could positively enhance the cells' longevity (and hence organisms).

Intermittent fasting may also play a key role in preventing cancer recurrence in women who had already been treated for cancer. Most times, these recurrences become more severe. Some cases of recurrence include stage IV breast cancer having a metastatic recurrence.

A study shows that women who carry out intermittent fasting exercise are less vulnerable to cancer recurrence (with a percentage of less than 36%). Intermittent fasting limits the amount of food that enters the body and reduces the amount of energy available to the cell.

Cells that are engaged in frequent restriction of Calories are known to less likely to develop changes that could lead to cancer. All these are owed to the positive and therapeutic effects of intermittent fasting on the cell and the immune system.

<u>Reduces Cardiovascular Disease</u>

Cardiovascular diseases (CVD) are known to have a very high mortality rate in women. Some of this CVD include; atherosclerotic cardiovascular disease (ASCVD), acute coronary syndrome (ACS), coronary artery disease (CAD), ischemic heart disease (IHD), etc.

Women above 50 have a higher chance of developing CVD, and although CVD affects both men and women, some risk factors increase the chances in women. These factors can be divided into two categories; modifiable and unmodifiable factors.

Among the unmodifiable factors are age, genetics, and gender. While the modifiable factors include hypertension, smoking, lack of physical exercise, obesity, poor diet, lipid metabolism disorder, diabetes, etc. Diabetes in women tends to increase the chances of a subtle heart attack without their knowledge.

Uncontrolled weight gain is the primary cause of obesity, which could lead to health disorders like diabetes, which increases the chances of developing CVD. Intermittent fasting has a great role it plays in insulin reduction, balancing heart rate, balancing high and low-density lipoprotein

Cholesterol (HDL and LDL). Also, it affects glucose levels as well as triglycerides, oxidative stress, and systemic inflammation.

Intermittent fasting boosts parasympathetic tone, which increases the variability of the heart rate. It does not only promote cardio-protection in overweight persons by enhancing weight loss; it works just as effectively in normal-weight individuals.

In other, for these positive changes to be lasting, one must continuously practice intermittently fasting, and the pattern or type of IF could depend on the preference of the individual.

Slows Down Aging Process

This is another benefit of intermittent fasting, and not until very recent years, the focus of intermittent fasting was to increase life span. This is because intermittent fasting was found to boost the body's general health and rejuvenate the body. The natural or even the induced aging process of the entire body is slowed down by doing this.

So, for women at 50 who, due to child-bearing and menopause, tend to age quicker than men, they can rely on strict adherence to intermittent fasting to slow down this process. The level of the effects of intermittent fasting varies from individual to individual.

However, its success is largely dependent on sex, age, genetic makeup, diet, environment, and other factors. Studies have shown that individuals who started intermittent fasting at a very young age have an increased lifespan (up to about 45%).

Individuals following a type of intermittent fasting experience strictly have a huge decrease in developing disorders that would be detrimental to their health. Hypertension, inflammation, obesity, dyslipidemia, and others, are lessened as a result of intermittent fasting. In fact, intermittent fasting is believed to have greater effects, which cannot be ascribed to only the reduction of calories.

Intermittent Fasting for Better Mental and Memory Performance

Intermittent fasting also enhances cognitive function and is very useful for boosting your brainpower. There are several factors of intermittent fasting, which can support this claim. First of all, it boosts the level of brain-derived neurotrophic factor (also known as BDNF), which is a protein in your brain that can interact with the parts of your brain responsible for controlling cognitive and memory functions as well as learning. BDNF can even protect and stimulate the growth of new brain cells.

Increase Physical Energy

This process influences not only your brain but also your digestive system. By setting a small feeding window and a larger fasting period, you will encourage the proper digestion of food. This leads to a proportional and healthy daily intake of food and calories. The more you get used to this process, the less you will experience hunger. If you are worried about slowing your metabolism, think again! Intermittent fasting enhances your metabolism; it makes metabolism more flexible, as the body now can run on glucose or fats for energy in a very effective way. In other words, intermittent fasting leads to better metabolism.

Oxygen use during exercise is a crucial part of the success of your training. You simply can't have performance without adjusting your breathing habits during workouts. VO2 max represents the maximum amount of oxygen your body can use per minute or kilogram of body weight. In popular terms, VO2 max is also referred to as "wind." The more oxygen you use, the better you will be able to perform. Top athletes can have twice the VO2 level of those without any training. A study focused on the VO2 levels of a fasted group (they just skipped breakfast) and a non-fasted group (they had breakfast an hour before). For both groups, the VO2 level was at 3.5 L/min at the beginning, and after the study, the level showed a significant increase of "wind" for the fasting group (9.7%), compared to just a 2.5% increase in the case of those with breakfast.

Increase Longevity

Autophagy is essential for the longevity of the organism. Autophagy has been shown to affect aging, which is why it plays such a large role in longevity. The reason for this is twofold. The first reason is that the cells that it acts in are often damaged or injured, and by way of autophagy, the disease or virus that is attempting to infect the organism is unable to spread, allowing the organism to continue living a relatively healthy life. This type of disease control increases the longevity of the organism.

The second reason is that autophagy is essential to maintaining the health of specific tissues and organs, which keeps them running smoothly and functioning at their best, which is also another factor that influences lifespan. If the organs and tissues are healthy, the organism as a whole will be healthy and will keep living.

In these two ways, autophagy plays a large role in the organisms' longevity and lifespan and their cells.

Autophagy can affect the quality of life of a person by maintaining their health and eliminating the disease. Inflammation in the short term helps to get rid of diseases, bacterial infections, and any sort of injury. By effectively eliminating disease and injury on time, the person's quality of life dramatically increases as their health is improved.

When it comes to the quality of life, autophagy has been shown to benefit mental health as well. Intermittent fasting, which induces autophagy, has been shown to decrease instances of depression and food-related disorders such as binge eating. Its benefits for weight loss also have been shown to improve body image, confidence, and overall self-satisfaction in adults who practice it for one month or more.

Other benefits of intermittent fasting include:

- Waistline reduction.

- Enhances psychological function.

- Prevention of neurodegenerative disorders, such as Parkinson's disease, stroke, etc.

- By reducing weight in obese women, intermittent fasting can dial down the symptoms of asthma.

- Tissue damages are reduced during intermittent fasting.

CHAPTER 3. INTERMITTENT FASTING FOR WOMEN OVER 50

According to researchers, intermittent fasting is beneficial for most people who eat during their daytime hours. Prolonged fasting differs from the usual eating style. If someone consumes 3 meals per day, including treats, and they don't work out, they operate on certain

Calories and don't burn their fat reserves at any time. Intermittent fasting allows our bodies to burn the reserved fat storage healthily; nine older women in ten have a form of chronic illness, and nearly eight in ten have more than one chronic disease. So, odds are, eventually, a person will get more. But to live a healthy life, there are measures one should take, and intermittent fasting is one of them.

Many of these chronic illnesses start from being overweight at an older age. The most important aspect of intermittent fasting is its weight loss assistance. Another research found that intermittent fasting induces less muscle loss than the more traditional form of daily restriction of calories. Bear in mind, though, that the primary explanation for its effectiveness is that intermittent fasting allows you to intake fewer calories overall. During your meal times, if you indulge and consume large quantities, you will not lose much weight at all.

Why Start Intermittent Fasting After 50?

Here, excess weight in women can cause these diseases, and intermittent fasting can help counteract them. Furthermore, intermittent fasting can help you control these aspects of living if you are over 50.

Hypertension

With age, blood vessels become less elastic when a person matures. This puts a strain on the mechanism that holds the body's blood. It may indicate why 2 in 3 women over the age of 50 have elevated blood pressure. The best approach to manage hypertension is to lose weight by intermittent fasting.

Diabetes

At least one in 10 women has diabetes. When you grow older, the odds of having the disease increase up. Heart failure, renal disease, blindness, and other complications may arise from diabetes due to excess weight.

Cardiac Condition

A significant source of heart attack is plaque formation in the arteries due to unhealthy eating. It begins in youth, and as one matures, it becomes worse. A large percentage of men and 5.6 percent of women have suffered from heart failure in the 40-58 age range in the U.S. Fasting and eating healthy is a good option to control any cardiovascular diseases.

Obesity

It might be dangerous for the health if one weighs too much for their height; it's not about getting a few extra pounds. More than 20 obesity chronic illnesses are correlated with stroke, asthma, arthritis, cancer, coronary failure, and high blood pressure. At least 30% of the older population is obese.

Arthritis

This condition of the joints was once directly attributed by physicians to the excessive wear and tear of time, and it sure is a cause. Yet biology and lifestyle are likely to have still much to do with it. A lack of physical exercise, diabetes, and becoming overweight may play a role in past joint accidents, too.

Osteoporosis

With old age, bones become weak, especially in women, which may lead to fractures. It impacts nearly 53.9 million Americans over 50 years of age. Some factors that will help: a balanced diet rich in vitamin D and calcium. Lose excess weight by fasting and daily weight-bearing activity, such as walking, jogging, and climbing stairs.

Tumor & Cancers

The greatest risk factor for old age is cancer. The disorder also impacts young adults, but between the ages of 46 and 54, your risk of getting it more than doubles. You can't influence a person's age or genes, but you have a choice in stuff like smoking or living an unhealthy lifestyle. With much of the study focusing on the beneficial impact that fasting has on cancer, fasting over varying periods has often helped older women decrease their risk of severe diseases. The study reported that fasting appears to suppress some cancer-causing pathways and can even delay tumor development.

Menopause

The classic indicators of menopause are hot flashes, insomnia, night sweats, mood swings, and vaginal dryness, burning, and itching. Heart failure and osteoporosis appear to escalate throughout the years of menopause. Often people start prolonged fasting to combat both the long-term and short-term symptoms of menopause. For several post-menopausal women, belly fat, not just for appearance but also for health, is a major concern. The decrease in belly fat resulting from intermittent fasting helped women minimize their likelihood of metabolic syndrome, a series of health conditions that enhance the risk of heart disease and diabetes for a post-menopausal female.

Advantages of Intermittent Fasting for Women Over 50

The benefits of intermittent fasting for women over 50 are limitless; some of them are mentioned here:

Decrease Insulin Resistance

Fasting is one of the most successful strategies to return the insulin receptors to a normal sensitivity level. Understanding the function of insulin plays is one of the biggest keys to learning about fasting and truly understanding every diet. About eating, insulin, the hormone that controls blood sugar, is formed in the pancreas and absorbed into the bloodstream. Insulin allows the body to retain energy as fat until released. Insulin creates fat because the fatter the body stores, the more insulin body makes or vice versa. The cycles during which a person is not eating allow the body time to reduce insulin levels, mainly during intermittent fasting, which changes the fat-storing mechanism. The mechanism goes in reverse, and the body loses weight as insulin levels decrease.

Autophagy is the amazing way cells "eat themselves" to get rid of dead cells and recycle younger parts. Autophagy is often the mechanism by which harmful pathogens, including viruses, bacteria, and other diseases, are killed. As the whole cell is recycled, another step in apoptosis. Your chance of cancer rises without this process when defective cells tend to multiply.

Intermittent Fasting Leads to Detoxification

Many of us have been subjected to contaminants from food and our climate in our lifetime. Many of these containments are processed in our bodies in fat cells. One of the most powerful methods to eliminate contaminants from the body is fasting and eating healthy.

The body's internal clock or Circadian Rhythm of the body controls virtually any mechanism in the body, and a chain of detrimental results will occur when it is disturbed. You adjust the circadian clock of the body while you take a rest from meals.

A Healthy Gut

It is one of the most important aspects of Fasting in that it provides a chance for the digestive tract and intestinal flora to reset. This is critical because the health of the body's digestive system regulates the immune system. There is even more proof that one's moods and emotional wellbeing are co-dependent on the gut microbiota. In recent studies of any area related to health and wellbeing, there has been a lot of hype on how one's gut flora might play an important part. The work of a more powerful immune system is important to a diverse microbiota, and it plays an important role in one's mental wellbeing. It also removes skin problems and reduces cancer danger.

Although the foods you consume have an immense effect on your intestinal health, periodic fasting in the digestive system can be another way to help grow the beneficial bacteria in the gut. Sugar and artificial goods disturb the equilibrium of your digestive tract between the beneficial and detrimental microbiota. Make sure to minimize packaged foods full of refined carbohydrates, sugars, and harmful fats that get the best outcome if you try intermittent fasting. Alternatively, switch to whole grains, plenty of organic vegetables and fruits, and good quality protein.

Intermittent fasting will work better by metabolic switching. Fasting contributes to lower glucose levels in the bloodstream. The body utilizes fat as an energy source instead of sugar after converting the fat into ketones.

Although it's not fasting, several physicians have recorded intermittent fasting advantages by permitting some easy-to-digest foods during the fasting window as fresh fruit. Modifications like this will also provide the essential rest for your metabolic and digestive system.

Losing Weight

It is expected that fasting helps accelerate the loss of excess weight. It also decreases insulin levels such that the body no longer receives the message to store more calories as fat during the state of fasting. Intermittent fasting may contribute to a self-activating decrease in calorie consumption by letting you consume fewer meals. Besides, to promote weight reduction, prolonged fasting affects hormone levels. It enhances noradrenaline or norepinephrine production, which is a fat-burning hormone, lowering insulin and rising growth hormone levels. Intermittent fasting can increase one's metabolic rate due to these changes in hormones. By encouraging one to eat less and activating ketones' production, intermittent fasting induces weight loss by adjusting all calorie calculation factors. In contrast to other weight loss trials, a study showed that this eating method would cause 3-8 percent weight loss in just weeks, which is a substantial percentage. People have lost 4 to 7 percent of their waist circumference; as per the same report, it is helpful for women dealing with menopause and unhealthy stomach fat that builds up over their organs and induces illness.

Other than insulin, during intermittent fasting are two important hormones, leptin and ghrelin. Ghrelin is the hormone of starvation that tells the body when it's hungry. Research shows intermittent fasting can reduce that ghrelin. There is also some evidence suggesting a rise in the leptin hormone, the hormone of satiety. That tells the body when it's full, and there's no more urge to eat.

People would be fuller quicker and hungry less frequently with less ghrelin and more leptin, which may lead to fewer calories eaten and, as a result, weight loss.

Tricks against Hunger Attacks

The best way to curb cravings is intermittent fasting. You don't eat for a certain number of hours each day, typically beginning at 6 am or later in this practice. You can have your main meal at noon and continue eating until 10 pm if you like, but it's generally recommended that you go without eating for 12-16 hours per day.

This practice of eating less often than normal and allowing your body to release stored sugar into your bloodstream is a proven method of curbing cravings and preventing hunger attacks. Intermittent fasting can also help curb the progress of aging, prevent heart disease, reduce cancer risk, and even boost immunity levels.

CHAPTER 4. INTERMITTENT FASTING TYPES

There are countless types of intermittent fasting. There are so many reasons why decide to follow an intermittent fasting lifestyle, and at least as many methods for doing it. Therefore, it is fundamental to set some basic definitions before we go deep in detail.

- Fasting – Giving up the intake of food or anything that has calories for a particular time frame. Normally, some non-caloric beverages and water are allowed.

- Intermittent Fasting – To fast intermittently by adding fasts into your regular meal plan.

- Extended Fasting – Fasting for a drawn-out time. It will, in general, be cultivated for a significant long time.

- Time-Restricted Feeding – Restricting your regular food usage inside a particular time window. This is meant to improve circadian rhythm and general wellness.

Generally, people who do intermittent fasting restrict their eating time and increase their fasting time. To have something like an actual fast, it would need to prop up for over 24 hours since that is the spot most of the benefits start to kick in.

First, let's have an overview of 10 of the main types of intermittent fasting, then we'll go deep into the 6 that better suit women after 50.

24-Hour Fasting

It is the fundamental technique of intermittent fasting—you fast for around 24 hours, and a short time later has a meal. Despite what the name may suggest, you won't actually go through an entire day without eating. Simply eat around the evening, fast all through the next day, and then eat again in the evening.

You can even have your food at the 23-hour check and eat it inside an hour. The idea is to make a very prominent caloric shortage for the day. Most of the benefits will be vain if you, regardless of fasting, binge and put on weight during the eating time frame.

Gradually and occasionally, you can decide to fast according to your physical condition and needs of the moment.

A fit person who works out constantly would require more eating time frames and a few fasting periods.

An overweight person who is sedentary and needs to lose some more weight could follow an intermittent fasting plan as long as they can until they lose the overabundance weight.

16/8 Intermittent Fasting

Martin Berkhan of Lean gains defined 16:8 intermittent fasting. It is used for improving fat loss while not having to go through an extremely demanding process.

You fast for 16 hours and eat your food inside 8. What number of meals you have inside that time length is irrelevant, yet whatever it is recommended to keep them around 2-3.

In my opinion, this should be the base fasting length to concentrate on reliably by everybody. There is no physical need to eat any sooner than that, and the restriction has many benefits.

Many people think it is more straightforward to postpone breakfast by two or three hours and then eat the last meal around early evening. You should not get insane, and it is demanding to observe the fast. The idea is simply to reduce the proportion of time we spend in an eating state and fast for a large portion of the day.

The Warrior Diet

Ori Hofmekler proposes the Warrior Diet. He talks about the benefits of fasting on blood pressure through hormesis.

The warrior diet not only improves your body's physical condition and resistance yet, moreover but also grows your mental attitude and outlook.

The Warrior Diet talks about old warriors like Spartans and Romans who used to remain on an empty stomach all through the day and eat in the evening. During daylight, they used to stroll around with 40 pounds of armor, build fortresses, and bear the hot sun of the Mediterranean, while having just a quick bite. They would have a huge supper around evening time consisting of stews, meat, bread, and many other things.

In the Warrior Diet, you fast for around 20 hours, have a short high power workout, and eat your food during a 4 hours window. Overall, it would merge either two minor meals with a break or one single huge supper.

One Meal a Day OMAD

One Meal a Day Diet, also called OMAD, simply consists of eating just one big meal every day

With OMAD, you regularly fast around 21-23 hours and eat your food inside a 1-2 hour time slot. This is remarkable for dieting since you can feel full and satisfied once the eating time comes.

It is unmatched for losing fat; be that as it may, not ideal for muscle improvement because of time for protein production and anabolism.

36-Hour Fasting

In the past, people would quite commonly go a couple of days without eating; they probably suffered and yet even thrived. Today, the average person can't bear to skip breakfast or go to bed hungry.

For over 24 hours is the spot where all the magic begins; the more you stay in a fasted state and experience hardship, the more your body is forced to trigger its supply systems that start to draw on fat stores, bolster rejuvenating microorganisms, and reuse old wrecked cell material through the system of autophagy.

It takes, at any rate, an entire day to see significant signs of autophagy. Yet, you can speed it up by eating low carb before starting the fast, rehearsing on an unfilled stomach, and drinking some homemade teas that facilitate the challenge.

For 36 hours, it's not really that annoying. You fundamentally eat the night before, don't eat anything during the day, go to sleep on an empty stomach, then wake up the next day, fast a few more hours, and begin eating again.

To make the fasting more straightforward, there are mineral water, plain coffee, green tea, and some homemade teas.

48-Hour Fasting

In case you made it to the 36-hour mark, why not give it a try to fast for a straight 48 hours.

It is only annoying getting through the change of habits. Once you overcome this obstacle, which generally occurs around your usual dinnertime, it gets a lot more straightforward.

The moment your body goes into an increasingly significant ketosis phase and autophagy starts, you will overcome hunger, feel very mentally clear, and have greater mindfulness and focus.

The most problematic bit of any complete fast is around the 24-hour mark. If you can make it to fall asleep and wake up the next day, you have set yourself prepared for fasting for a significant time with no issues from that moment onward. You essentially need to get over this hidden obstacle.

Going to bed hungry sounds disturbing; in any case, this is what a huge part of the world's population does daily. This could make you think about your own luck and feel thankful for having food anytime you want.

Expanded Fasting (3-7 Days)

48-hours fasting would give you a short ride in autophagy and some fat consumption. To genuinely get the deep health benefits of fasting, you would have to fast for three or more days.

It has been shown that 72-hours of fasting can reset the immune system in mice. However, studies on humans have not confirmed that conclusion; also, there may be some issues in prolonged fasting that are not under severe medical control.

Three to five days is the perfect time frame for autophagy, after which you may begin to see unwanted losses in bulk and muscle. Fasting for seven or more days is not generally suggested. Most people do not need to fast any longer than that since it may make them lose muscle tissue.

Fit people may want to focus on three-four of these expanded fasts every year, to propel cell recovery and clean out the body. Notwithstanding a healthy eating routine without any junk food, I do it anyway four times a year because of their tremendous benefits.

In case you are overweight or experience the negative effects of some illness, then longer fasts can really help you get back in health. Fast for three to five days, have a little refreshment break and repeat the plan until needed. I'll never say that enough; if you decide to go through this kind of longer fasting, be always sure of what you are doing and consult a doctor for any doubt.

Alternate Day Fasting

Alternate Day Fasting, as for the 5:2 Diet, is a very common type of fasting. Are they fully considered fasting, despite allowing the intake of 500/660 calories a day on fasting days? Well, yes, they are, since these limited amounts of calories are only intended to help extend perseverance.

To have a sporadic caloric intake will not enable the whole of the physiological benefits of fasting to fully manifest. It would limit a part of the effect. In any case, a strict limitation is important for both your physiology and mind.

Everybody can fast. It is just that someone cannot psychologically bear the weight of not eating. Fasting mimicking diets and alternate-day fasting in this respect.

Fasting Mimicking Diet (FMD)

The Fasting Mimicking Diet can be used every so often. Commonly, people who cannot actually fast, like old people or some recovering patients follow it.

Fasting mimicking diet has been shown to reduce blood pressure, lower insulin, and cover IGF-1, all of which have positive life length benefits. Regardless, these effects are likely an immediate consequence of the huge caloric restriction.

During the Fasting Mimicking Diet, you would eat low protein, moderate carb, and moderate fat foods like mushroom soup, olives, kale wafers, and some nut bars. The idea is to give you something to eat while keeping the calories as low as reasonable. In most cases, again, this is more about satisfying people's psychological needs of eating than the physical ones.

With zero calories would be just as effective, and it would keep up more muscle tissue by increasingly significant ketosis. To thwart the unwanted loss of lean mass, you can adapt the macronutrient taken in during Fasting Mimicking Diet and make them more ketogenic by cutting down the carbs and increasing the fats.

Protein Sparing Modified Fasting

Protein-Sparing Modified Fast (PSMF) is a low carb, low fat, high protein type of diet that helps to get increasingly fit quite fast while keeping muscle toned.

Lean mass is a significant matter of stress for healthy people, especially in case they are endeavoring to do intermittent fasting.

A catabolic stressor will, over the long term, lead to muscle loss; notwithstanding, the loss rate is a lot lower than people may imagine. To prevent that from happening, you have to stay in ketosis and lower the body's appetite for glucose.

PSMF is absolutely going to keep up more muscle than the fasting-mimicking diet. Yet, there's the danger of staying out of ketosis in case you are already eating many proteins preparing yourself for muscle catabolism.

CHAPTER 5. BREAKFASTS

1. <u>Greek-Style Frittata with Spinach and Feta Cheese</u>

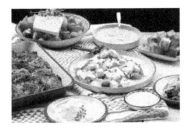

Preparation Time: 10 minutes

Cooking Time: 3.5-4 hours on low

Servings: 6

Ingredients:

- 2 cups of spinach, fresh or frozen

- 6 eggs, lightly beaten

- 1 cup of plain yogurt

- 1 small onion, cut into small pieces

- 2 red roasted peppers, peeled

- 1 garlic clove, crushed

- 1 cup of feta cheese, crumbled

- 2 Tablespoons of softened butter

- 2 Tablespoons of olive oil

- Salt and pepper to taste

- 1 teaspoon of dried oregano

Directions:

1. Sauté the onion and garlic for 5 minutes. Add the spinach, heat for an additional 2 minutes. Let the mixture cool down.

2. Roast the red peppers in a dry pan or under the broiler. Peel them and cut them into small pieces. You can use roasted peppers from a jar, but use those without vinegar.

3. In a separate bowl, beat the eggs, yogurt, and seasoning. Combine well.

4. Add the peppers and the onion mixture. Mix again.

5. Crumble the feta cheese with a fork and add it to the frittata.

6. Grease the bottom and sides of the Slow Cooker with butter. Pour the mixture in.

7. Cover, cook on low for 3.5-4 hours.

Nutrition:

- Calories 312 kcal Carbohydrates 9 g Protein 18 g

- Fiber 25 g

2. Avocado Smoothie

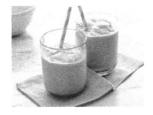

Preparation Time: 5 minutes

Cooking Time: 0 minutes

Servings: 4

Ingredients:

- 1 whole avocado

- 1 ounce of chopped mint

- 1 glass of water 1 ounce of berries

- 2 ounces of heavy cream (20%)

- 1 tablespoon of cocoa powder (optional)

- Cinnamon and stevia to taste

Directions:

1. Weigh all food on a measuring scale.

2. Remove the pit and skin from the avocado.

3. Cut the mint into small pieces for your blender.

4. Place the remaining ingredients in the blender and blend at high speed for about 30 seconds to the desired consistency.

Tip: This smoothie has 19 grams of pure fiber, so there are 20 grams of net carbs. Remember that carbohydrates fiber equals net carbohydrates. If you're worried about Keto proportions, try removing the recipe's berries and adding more cream.

Nutrition:

- Calories 515 kcal

- Fat 43 g

- Protein 8 g

- Net carbs 20 g

3. <u>Turmeric Muffins</u>

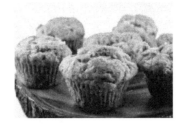

Preparation Time: 10 minutes

Cooking Time: 23 minutes

Servings: 6

Ingredients:

- 2 cups of almond flour

- ½ cup of powdered Erythritol

- 3 scoops of turmeric tonic

- 1½ teaspoons of organic baking powder

- 3 organic eggs

- 1 cup of mayonnaise

- ½ teaspoon of organic vanilla extract

Directions:

1. Preheat your oven to 350 °F.

2. Line a 12 cups muffin tin with paper liners.

3. In a large bowl, add flour, Erythritol, turmeric tonic, and baking powder, and mix well.

4. Add the eggs, mayonnaise, and vanilla extract, and beat until well combined.

5. Place the mixture into the prepared muffin cups evenly.

6. Bake for approximately 20–23 minutes or until a toothpick inserted in the center comes out clean.

7. Remove the muffin tin from the oven and place it onto a wire rack to cool for about 10 minutes.

8. Carefully invert the muffins onto the wire rack to cool completely before serving.

Nutrition:

- Calories 516 kcal Net Carbs 3.9 g Total Fat 48.9 g

- Saturated Fat 6 g Cholesterol 95 mg Sodium 272 mg

- Total Carbs 8 g Fiber 4.1 g Sugar 1.9 g Protein 2.8 g

4. Kale, Edamame and Tofu Curry

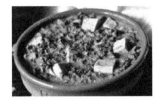

Preparation Time: 20 minutes

Cooking Time: 40 minutes

Servings: 3

Ingredients:

- 1 tablespoon of rapeseed oil

- 1 large onion, chopped

- 4 cloves of garlic, peeled and grated

- 1 large thumb (7cm) of fresh ginger, peeled and grated

- 1 red chili, deseeded and thinly sliced

- 1/2 teaspoon of ground turmeric

- 1/4 teaspoon of cayenne pepper

- 1 teaspoon of paprika

- 1/2 teaspoon of ground cumin

- 1 teaspoon of salt

- 250 g / 9 ounces of dried red lentils

- 1-liter of boiling water

- 50 g / 1.7 ounces of frozen soya beans

- 200 g / 7 ounces of firm tofu, chopped into cubes

- 2 tomatoes, roughly chopped

- Juice of 1 lime

- 200 g / 7 ounces of kale leaves stalk removed and torn

Directions:

1. Put the oil in a pan over low heat. Add your onion and cook for 5 minutes before adding the garlic, ginger, and chili and cooking for a further 2 minutes. Add your turmeric, cayenne, paprika, cumin, and salt and Stir through before adding the red lentils and stirring again.

2. Pour in the boiling water and allow it to simmer for 10 minutes, reduce the heat and cook for about 20-30 minutes until the curry has a thick 'porridge' consistency.

3. Add your tomatoes, tofu, and soya beans and cook for a further 5 minutes. Add your kale leaves, lime juice, and cook until the kale is just tender.

Nutrition:

- Calories 133 kcal

- Carbohydrate 54 g

- Protein 43 g

5. <u>Baked Eggs</u>

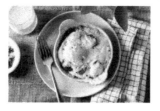

Preparation Time: 10 minutes

Cooking Time: 12 minutes

Servings: 4

Ingredients:

- 4 tablespoons of half-and-half heavy cream

- 4 organic eggs

- ½ ounce of Gruyere cheese, shredded

- Salt and ground black pepper, to taste

- 4 teaspoons of fresh chives, minced

Directions:

1. Preheat your oven to 375 °F.

2. Grease 4 ramekins.

3. In the bottom of each prepared ramekin, place 1 tablespoon of the heavy cream.

4. Carefully, crack 1 egg into each ramekin and sprinkle with the cheese, followed by salt, black pepper, and chives.

5. Bake for approximately 8–12 minutes until the desired doneness of the eggs.

6. Serve hot.

Nutrition:

- Calories 97 kcal

- Net Carbs 1 g

- Total Fat 7.3 g Saturated Fat 3.1 g

- Cholesterol 173 mg Sodium 118 mg

- Total Carbs 1 g

- Fiber 0 g

- Sugar 0.4 g

- Protein 7.1 g

6. <u>Tofu & Mushroom Muffins</u>

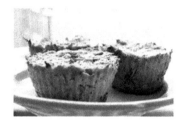

Preparation Time: 15 minutes

Cooking Time: 30 minutes

Servings: 6

Ingredients:

- 1 teaspoon of olive oil

- 1½ cup of fresh mushrooms, chopped

- 1 scallion, chopped

- 1 teaspoon of garlic, minced

- 1 teaspoon of fresh rosemary, minced

- Freshly ground black pepper, to taste

- 1 (12.3-ounce) of package lite firm silken tofu, drained

- ¼ cup of unsweetened almond milk

- 2 tablespoons of Parmesan cheese, grated

- 1 tablespoon of arrowroot starch

- 1 teaspoon of butter, softened

- ¼ teaspoon of ground turmeric

Directions:

1. Preheat your oven to 375 °F.

2. Grease 12 cups of muffin tin.

3. In a non-stick skillet, heat the oil over medium heat and sauté the scallion and garlic for about 1 minute.

4. Add the mushrooms and sauté for about 5–7 minutes.

5. Stir in the rosemary and black pepper and remove from the heat

6. Set aside to cool slightly.

7. In a food processor, add the tofu and the remaining ingredients and pulse until smooth.

8. Transfer the tofu mixture into a large bowl.

9. Fold in the mushroom mixture.

10. Place the mixture into the prepared muffin cups evenly.

11. Bake for approximately 20–22 minutes or until a toothpick inserted in the center comes out clean.

12. Remove the muffin pan from the oven and place it onto a wire rack to cool for about 10 minutes.

13. Carefully invert the muffins onto a wire rack and serve warm.

Nutrition:

- Calories 63

- Net Carbs2.3 g

- Total Fat 3.6 g

- Saturated Fat: 1 g

- Cholesterol 3 mg

- Sodium 49 mg

- Total Carbs 2.8 g

- Fiber 0.5 g

- Sugar 1.1 g

- Protein 5.4 g

7. <u>MCT Protein Smoothie</u>

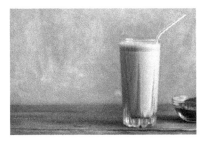

Preparation Time: 5 minutes

Cooking Time: 0 minutes

Servings: 1

Ingredients:

- 1 cup of almond or coconut milk

- 1 scoop of whey protein powder (preferably keto-friendly protein)

- 1 scoop of MCT powder (or 1-2 tsp. of MCT oil)

- ½ teaspoon of cinnamon

- Cocoa powder and stevia to taste

Directions:

1. Add all the ingredients to a high-speed blender and blend until smooth.

2. If you love iced smoothies, add ice!

Tip: not all proteins are keto-friendly. When buying, be sure to look at the ingredients. Avoid industrial sweeteners. I use a protein that contains stevia. You can find that too.

Nutrition:

- Calories 231 kcal

- Fat 12 g

- Protein 25 g

- Carbs 4 g

8. <u>Bell Pepper Frittata</u>

Preparation Time: 15 minutes

Cooking Time: 10 minutes

Servings: 6

Ingredients:

- 8 organic eggs

- 1 tablespoon of fresh cilantro, chopped

- 1 tablespoon of fresh basil, chopped

- ¼ teaspoon of red pepper flakes, crushed

- Salt and ground black pepper, to taste

- 2 tablespoons of unsalted butter

- 1 bunch of scallions, chopped

- 1 cup of bell pepper, seeded and sliced thinly

- ½ cup of goat cheese, crumbled

Directions:

1. Preheat the broiler of the oven.

2. Arrange a rack in the upper third of the oven.

3. In a bowl, add the eggs, fresh herbs, red pepper flakes, salt, and black pepper, and beat well.

4. In an ovenproof skillet, melt the butter over medium heat and sauté the scallion and bell pepper for about 1 minute.

5. Add the egg mixture over bell pepper mixture evenly and lift the edges to let the egg mixture flow underneath and cook for about 2–3 minutes.

6. Place the cheese on top in the form of dots.

7. Now, transfer the skillet under broiler and broil for about 2–3 minutes.

8. Remove from the oven and set aside for about 5 minutes before serving.

9. Cut the frittata into desired-sized slices and serve.

Nutrition:

- Calories 183 kcalNet Carbs 0 g Total Fat 14.4 g

- Saturated Fat 7.3 g Cholesterol 248 mg Sodium 338 mg

- Total Carbs 2.3 g Fiber 0.4 g Sugar 1 g Protein 11.7 g

9. Peanut Keto Smoothie

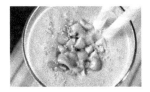

Preparation Time: 5 minutes

Cooking Time: 0 minutes

Servings: 1

Ingredients:

- 1/2 cup of almond milk (unsweetened)

- 1 tablespoon of nut butter (peanut butter, walnut oil) can be substituted for coconut oil

- 1 tablespoon of cocoa powder (preferably organic)

- 2 tablespoons of roasted peanuts (salted)

- 1/4 medium avocado

- Stevia to taste, mint, and ice of your choice

Directions:

1. Weigh all the ingredients. Then add to a blender or food processor.

2. Mix it well.

3. If the smoothie is too thick, you can add a little milk to change the consistency.

4. If the smoothie is too runny, you can add more cocoa powder or peanuts.

Tip: this should be consumed immediately after preparation, but if you decide to enjoy it later then stir well before drinking as it may come off.

Nutrition:

- Calories 216 kcal

- Fat 17 g

- Protein 6 g

- Carbs 8 g

10. Keto Berry Smoothie

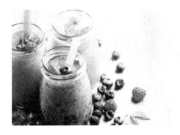

Preparation Time: 5 minutes

Cooking Time: 0 minutes

Servings: 4

Ingredients:

- 1 cup of unsweetened coconut milk

- 1 cup of berries (blackberries, blueberries, strawberries, raspberries), frozen or fresh of your choice

- 2 scoops of keto protein (replace with coconut or almond flour)

- 2 tablespoons of heavy cream

- Stevia to taste, mint, and ice of your choice

Directions:

1. Add all the ingredients to a blender.

2. Mix well.

3. If using ice, add this and stir again.

4. Beat until the consistency you want.

Tip: it should be consumed immediately. If you want to save this for later, mix well before use. Add more heavy cream to this smoothie to make it more nutritious.

Nutrition:

- Calories 114 kcal

- Fat 7 g

- Protein 7 g

- Carbs 5 g

11. Mayonnaise Waffles

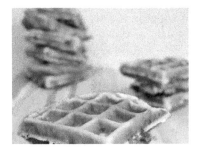

Preparation Time: 15 minutes

Cooking Time: 10 minutes

Servings: 2

Ingredients:

- ½ cup of blanched almond flour

- 2 tablespoons of Erythritol

- ½ teaspoon of organic baking powder

- ¼ teaspoon of salt

- 1 large organic egg (separated)

- ¼ cup of unsweetened almond milk

- 2 tablespoons of butter, melted

- 2 tablespoons of almond butter, melted

- ½ teaspoon of organic vanilla extract

Directions:

1. In a large bowl, mix the almond flour, Erythritol, baking powder, and salt.

2. In a second clean glass bowl, add the egg white and beat until stiff peaks form. Set aside.

3. In a third bowl, add egg yolks, almond milk, butter, almond butter, and vanilla extract and beat until well combined.

4. Add the flour mixture and mix until smooth.

5. Gently, fold in the whipped egg whites.

6. Preheat the waffle iron and then grease it.

7. Place ½ of the mixture into preheated waffle iron and cook for about 4–5 minutes or until golden-brown.

8. Repeat with the remaining mixture.

9. Serve warm.

Nutrition:

- Calories 425 kcal

- Net Carbs 4.4 g

- Total Fat 38.5 g

- Saturated Fat 9.8 g

- Cholesterol 124 mg

- Sodium 134 mg

- Total Carbs 9.2 g

- Fiber 4.8 g

- Sugar 2 g

- Protein 6.8 g

12. <u>Bacon Omelet</u>

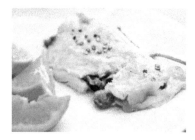

Preparation Time: 15 minutes

Cooking Time: 15 minutes

Servings: 2

Ingredients:

- 4 large organic eggs

- 1 tablespoon of fresh chives, minced

- Salt and ground black pepper, to taste

- 4 bacon slices 1 tablespoon of unsalted butter

- 2 ounces of cheddar cheese, shredded

Directions:

1. In a bowl, add the eggs, chives, salt, and black pepper, and beat until well combined.

2. Heat a non-stick frying pan over medium-high heat and cook the bacon slices for about 8–10 minutes.

3. Place the bacon onto a paper towel-lined plate to drain. Then chop the bacon slices.

4. With paper towels, wipe out the frying pan.

5. In the same frying pan, melt the butter over medium-low heat and cook the egg mixture for about 2 minutes.

6. Carefully flip the omelet and top with chopped bacon.

7. Cook for 1–2 minutes or until the desired doneness of eggs.

8. Remove from heat and immediately place the cheese in the center of the omelet.

9. Fold the edges of the omelet over the cheese and cut into 2 portions.

10. Serve immediately.

Nutrition:

- Calories 622 kcal Net Carbs 2 g Total Fat 49.3 g Saturated Fat 20.7 g Cholesterol 481 mg Sodium 1,600 mg Total Carbs 2 g

- Fiber 0 g Sugar: 1 g Protein 41.2 g

13. Antipasti Skewers

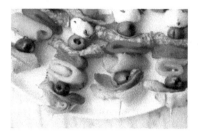

Preparation Time: 10 minutes

Cooking Time: 0 minute

Servings: 6

Ingredients:

- 6 small mozzarella balls

- 1 tablespoon of olive oil

- Salt to taste

- 1/8 teaspoon of dried oregano

- 2 roasted yellow peppers, sliced into strips and rolled

- 6 cherry tomatoes

- 6 green olives, pitted

- 6 Kalamata olives, pitted

- 2 artichoke hearts, sliced into wedges

- 6 slices salami, rolled

- 6 leaves fresh basil

Directions:

1. Toss the mozzarella balls in olive oil.

2. Season with salt and oregano.

3. Thread the mozzarella balls and the rest of the ingredients into skewers.

4. Serve in a platter.

Nutrition:

- Calories 180 kcal Total Fat 11.8 g

- Saturated Fat 4.5 g Cholesterol 26 mg

- Sodium 482 mg Total Carbohydrate 11.7 g

- Dietary Fiber 4.8 g Total Sugars 4.1 g

- Protein 9.2 g Potassium 538 mg

14. Chocolate Cupcakes with Matcha Icing

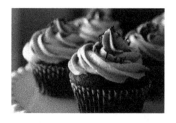

Preparation Time: 35 minutes

Cooking Time: 0 minutes

Servings: 4

Ingredients:

- 150g / 5 ounces of self-rising flour

- 200 g / 7 ounces of caster sugar

- 60 g / 2.1 ounces of cocoa

- ½ teaspoon of salt

- ½ teaspoon of fine espresso coffee, decaf if preferred

- 120 ml / ½ cup of milk

- ½ teaspoon of vanilla extract

- 50 ml / ¼ cup of vegetable oil

- 1 egg

- 120 ml / ½ cup of water

For the icing:

- 50 g / 1.7 ounces of butter

- 50 g / 1.7 ounces of icing sugar

- 1 tablespoon of matcha green tea powder

- ½ teaspoon of vanilla bean paste

- 50 g / 1.7 ounces of soft cream cheese

Directions:

1. Heat the oven and line a cupcake tin with paper.

2. Put the flour, sugar, cocoa, salt, and coffee powder in a large bowl and mix well.

3. Add milk, vanilla extract, vegetable oil, and egg to dry ingredients, and use an electric mixer to beat until well combined. Gently pour the boiling water slowly and beat on low speed until completely combined. Use the high speed to beat for another minute to add air to the dough. The dough is much

more liquid than a normal cake mix. Have faith; It will taste fantastic!

4. Arrange the dough evenly between the cake boxes. Each cake box must not be more than ¾ full. Bake for 15-18 minutes, until the dough resumes when hit. Remove from oven and allow cooling completely before icing.

5. To make the icing, beat your butter and icing sugar until they turn pale and smooth. Add the matcha powder and vanilla and mix again. Add the cream cheese and beat until it is smooth. Pipe or spread on the cakes.

Nutrition:

- Calories 435 kcal

- Fat 5 g

- Fiber 3 g

- Carbs 7 g

- Protein 9 g

15. <u>Sesame Chicken Salad</u>

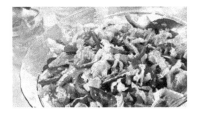

Preparation Time: 20 minutes

Cooking Time: 0 minutes **Servings:** 4

Ingredients:

- 1 tablespoon of sesame seeds

- 1 cucumber, peeled, halved lengthwise, without a teaspoon, and sliced

- 100 g / 3.5 ounces of black cabbage, chopped

- 60 g of pak choi, finely chopped

- ½ red onion, thinly sliced

- Large parsley (20 g / 0.7 ounces), chopped

- 150 g / 5 ounces of cooked chicken, minced

<u>For the dressing:</u>

- 1 tablespoon of extra virgin olive oil

- 1 teaspoon of sesame oil 1 lime juice 1 teaspoon of light honey

- 2 teaspoons of soy sauce

Directions:

1. Roast your sesame seeds in a dry pan for 2 minutes until they become slightly golden and fragrant.

2. Transfer to a plate to cool.

3. In a small bowl, mix olive oil, sesame oil, lime juice, honey, and soy sauce to prepare the dressing.

4. Place the cucumber, black cabbage, pak choi, red onion, and parsley in a large bowl and mix gently.

5. Pour over the dressing and mix again.

6. Distribute the salad between two dishes and complete with the shredded chicken. Sprinkle with sesame seeds just before serving.

Nutrition:

- Calories 345 kcal Fat 5 g Fiber 2 g

- Carbs 10 g Protein 4 g

16. Jalapeno Poppers

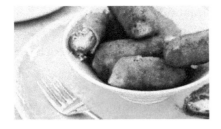

Preparation Time: 30 minutes

Cooking Time: 60 minutes

Servings: 10

Ingredients:

- 5 fresh jalapenos, sliced and seeded

- 4 ounces of package cream cheese

- ¼ pound of bacon, sliced in half

Directions:

1. Preheat your oven to 275 ° F.

2. Place a wire rack over your baking sheet.

3. Stuff each jalapeno with cream cheese and wrap it in bacon.

4. Secure with a toothpick.

5. Place on the baking sheet.

6. Bake for 1 hour and 15 minutes.

Nutrition:

- Calories 103 kcal

- Total Fat 8.7 g

- Saturated Fat 4.1 g

- Cholesterol 25 mg

- Sodium 296 mg

- Total Carbohydrate 0.9 g

- Dietary Fiber 0.2 g

- Total Sugars 0.3 g

- Protein 5.2 g

- Potassium 93 mg

17. <u>Vanilla Smoothie</u>

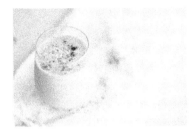

Preparation Time: 5 minutes

Cooking Time: 0 minutes

Servings: 2

Ingredients:

- 1 tablespoon of organic vanilla extract

- 3–4 drops of liquid stevia

- 1 cup of heavy cream

- 1 1/3 cups of unsweetened almond milk

- ¼ cup of ice cubes

Directions:

1. In a high-speed blender, put all the ingredients and pulse until creamy.

2. Pour the smoothie into two glasses and serve immediately.

Nutrition:

- Calories 252 kcal

- Net Carbs 0 g

- Total Fat 24.5 g

- Saturated Fat 14 g

- Cholesterol 82 mg

- Sodium 143 mg

- Total Carbs 3.8 g

- Fiber 0.7 g

- Sugar 0.9 g

- Protein 1.9 g

18. <u>Turmeric Smoothie</u>

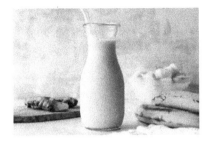

Preparation Time: 10 minutes

Cooking Time: 0 minutes

Servings: 2

Ingredients:

- 2 tablespoons of chia seeds

- 1 tablespoon of ground turmeric

- 1 teaspoon of ground cinnamon

- 2 tablespoons of MCT oil 2 teaspoons of stevia powder

- 1¾ cups of unsweetened almond milk ¼ cup of ice cubes

Directions:

1. In a high-speed blender, put all the ingredients and pulse until creamy.

2. Pour the smoothie into two glasses and serve immediately.

Nutrition:

- Calories 179 kcal

- Net Carbs 3.2 g

- Total Fat 19.9 g

- Saturated Fat 14.6 g

- Cholesterol 0 mg

- Sodium 159 mg

- Total Carbs 7.9 g

- Fiber 4.7 g

- Sugar 0.1 g

- Protein 2.7 g

19. Coffee Smoothie

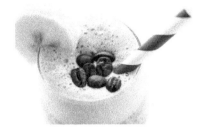

Preparation Time: 10 minutes

Cooking Time: 0 minutes

Servings: 2

Ingredients:

- 1 cup of brewed coffee

- 2 tablespoons of MCT oil

- 1 teaspoon of vanilla extract

- 1/8 teaspoon of stevia powder

- 1 cup of heavy cream 1 cup of ice cubes

Directions:

1. In a high-speed blender, put all the ingredients and pulse until creamy.

2. Pour the smoothie into two glasses and serve immediately.

Nutrition:

- Calories 314 kcal

- Net Carbs 1.9 g

- Total Fat 36.2 g

- Saturated Fat 27.8 g

- Cholesterol 82 mg

- Sodium 29 mg

- Total Carbs 1.9 g

- Fiber 0 g

- Sugar0.3 g

- Protein 1.4 g

CHAPTER 6. LUNCH

20. Baked Mushrooms with Pumpkin and Chipotle Polenta

Preparation Time: 15 minutes

Cooking Time: 40 minutes **Servings:** 3

Ingredients:

- 900 g mix of mushrooms, chopped

- 1/3 cup of extra virgin oil

- 1 garlic head, crushed cloves

- A small handful of sage, finely chopped or sliced

- Sea salt and freshly ground black pepper.

- 1 cup of cooked pumpkin puree

- 3 cups of chicken broth Nutmeg, freshly grated

- 1 chipotle adobo sauce, seedless and finely chopped, plus a small spoon of adobo sauce

- 1 cup of quick-cooking polenta

- 2 tablespoons of butter

- 2 tablespoons of honey

- Roasted seeds for decoration

- Chives, minced, for decoration

Directions:

1. Warm your oven to 220 °C. Mix the mushrooms with extra virgin olive oil, garlic, brine, salt, plus pepper, and bake within 25 minutes.

2. Meanwhile, in a small pan, put it pumpkin puree over medium heat, along with some chicken broth to dilute—season with salt, pepper, and nutmeg.

3. Put the remaining stock and bring to a boil in another pan, then add the chipotle, adobo sauce, polenta, and mix using a wire whisk.

4. Continue beating the polenta until the sides are far from the pan walls, then add the butter, honey, and beat again.

5. Combine pumpkin and polenta and serve in individual shallow bowls. Top with roasted mushrooms and Siva with roasted seeds and chives for garnish.

Nutrition:

- Calories 151 kcal Protein 7.1 g Carbs 6.7 g

- Fat 10.9 g Phosphorus 44 mg Potassium 121.8 mg

- Sodium 256.6 mg

21. Quinoa Salad with Chickpeas and Feta

Preparation Time: 15 minutes

Cooking Time: 15 minutes

Servings: 4

Ingredients:

- 1 onion, chopped

- 1 toe garlic, chopped

- 1 tablespoon of olive oil

- 150 ml vegetable broth

- 100 g of Quinoa 60 g of Feta

- 215 g of (Drained weight, from the jar) chickpeas

- 1 small bunch of coriander

- 1/2 lemon Salt Pepper

- 1/2 teaspoon of Ras el Hanout

Directions:

1. Sauté the onion plus garlic in a saucepan with oil. Deglaze using the vegetable stock, bring to the boil and cook the quinoa according to the instructions on the packet.

2. In the meantime, pour the chickpeas out of the glass into a sieve, rinse and drain. Wash the coriander, shake dry and chop.

3. Squeeze the lemon. Prepare a dressing from lemon juice, salt, pepper, Ras el Hanout, and coriander. Put the finished quinoa in a bowl, pour the drained chickpeas and the dressing over it.

4. Finally, crumble the feta and mix it with the quinoa salad. Let it steep for at least 15 minutes. The salad tastes lukewarm or cold.

Nutrition:

- Calories 469 kcal

- Protein 20 g

- Fat 20 g

- Carbohydrates 52 g

- Phosphorus 526 mg

- Potassium 445.9 mg

- Sodium 384.8 mg

22. Green Asparagus Soup

Preparation Time: 15 minutes

Cooking Time: 30 minutes

Servings: 2

Ingredients:

- 250 g of green asparagus

- 1 shallot

- 10 g of butter (1 tbsp)

- 400 ml of classic vegetable broth

- 30 g of parmesan (1 piece)

- ½ lemon

- 4 tablespoons of soy cream salt pepper

- 100 ml of milk (1.5% fat)

- 3 drops of truffle oil

Directions:

1. Wash and drain the asparagus and cut off any woody ends. Peel the asparagus in the lower third. Cut the sticks into pieces about 2 cm long. Peel and finely chop the shallot.

2. Heat the butter in a saucepan. Sauté the asparagus pieces and shallot in it over medium heat. Put in the vegetable stock and boil on low heat for about 15 minutes.

3. Meanwhile, finely grate the Parmesan cheese, add it to the asparagus and blend finely with a hand blender.

4. Squeeze the lemon. Stir the soy cream into the soup, season with salt, pepper, and a little lemon juice.

5. Heat the milk, add a pinch of salt and the truffle oil (about 140°F), and do not let it boil. Beat the milk until frothy with a hand mixer.

6. Pour the soup into glasses or glass cups; distribute the milk foam on top. Serve immediately.

Nutrition:

- Calories 197 kcal

- Protein 10 g

- Fat 14 g

- Carb 6 g

- Phosphorus 0 mg

- Potassium 368 mg

- Sodium 198 mg

23. <u>Potato Salad with Asparagus</u>

Preparation Time: 15 minutes

Cooking Time: 30 minutes

Servings: 4

Ingredients:

- 500 g of mainly waxy potatoes

- salt

- 500 g of green asparagus

- 5 tomatoes, sliced into wedges

- 1 handful chervil, chopped

- 200 ml of vegetable broth

- 2 tablespoons of rapeseed oil

- 4 tablespoons of vinegar

- pepper

- 4 large lettuce leaves for garnish

Directions:

1. Wash the potatoes thoroughly and cook them for about 20 minutes in salted water.

2. In the meantime, wash the asparagus, peel, and cut off the lower third's hard ends. Cut the sticks into pieces diagonally, approx. Length: 3 cm.

3. Cook for approximately 8 minutes in boiling salted water, then drain, rinse in cold water and drain.

4. Put aside about 4 stalks for garnish. Drain the potatoes when the cooking time is over, rinse them, and peel them while they are still hot.

5. Cut the potatoes into slices and pour over them with the hot stock. Mix in the tomatoes, asparagus, and chervil. Add oil and vinegar to the salad, salt, pepper, and season to taste.

6. Wash the leaves of the lettuce, shake them dry, and spread them over the bowls. Arrange the asparagus on top with the potato salad. Add the chervil to the garnish and serve.

Nutrition:

- Calories 178 kcal Protein 6 g

- Fat 5 g Carbohydrates 25 g

- Phosphorus 55 mg

- Potassium 235.8 mg

- Sodium 452.6 mg

24. <u>Chicken and Asparagus Salad with Watercress</u>

Preparation Time: 15 minutes

Cooking Time: 5 minutes

Servings: 4

Ingredients:

- 100 g of spring onions, cut into thin rings

- 200 g of cherry tomatoes, quartered

- 100 g of green asparagus, thin slices

- 600 g of chicken breast fillet (4 chicken breast fillets)

- salt

- pepper

- 1 small lime

- 1 clove of garlic

- 6 tablespoons of honey

- 1 tablespoon of grainy mustard

- 5 tablespoons of olive oil

- 100 g of watercress

Directions:

1. Wash the chicken fillets, pat dry with kitchen paper, and cut into strips. Season with salt and pepper. For the dressing, cut the lime in half and squeeze out the juice.

2. Peel and dice the garlic. Mix with honey, mustard, 3 tablespoons of lime juice, and 3 tablespoons of oil—season with salt and pepper. Warm-up the rest of the oil in a large non-stick pan and stir-fry the meat for about 5 minutes over high heat.

3. Put the chicken, spring onions, tomatoes, and asparagus in a bowl. Mix in the dressing and let the salad steep for about 10 minutes.

4. In the meantime, wash the watercress and shake dry. Pluck the leaves, coarsely chop as desired, and distribute on plates or bowls. Flavor the chicken salad with salt and pepper and serve on the cress.

Nutrition:

- Calories 633 kcal Protein 37 g

- Fat 14 g Carbohydrates 22 g

- Potassium 450 mg

- Sodium 640 mg

- Phosphorus 0 mg

25. Chicken and Zucchini Salad with Nuts

Preparation Time: 15 minutes

Cooking Time: 15 minutes

Servings: 4

Ingredients:

- 3 zucchinis, sliced

- 500 g of chicken breast fillet

- salt

- pepper

- 4 tablespoons of olive oil

- ½ fret mint

- ½ lemon

- 80 g of pecans

Directions:

1. Season the zucchini with salt and pepper. Rinse the chicken fillet under cold water, and pat dry.

2. In a pan, heat 2 tablespoons of oil. Fry the chicken in it for approximately 10 minutes over medium heat until golden

brown. Reduce the heat and let the fillets of the chicken breast cook.

3. In another pan, heat the remaining oil. Sauté slices of zucchini in it for about 4 minutes over medium heat.

4. Wash the mint, shake the dry leaves, and pluck them. Squeeze the lemons in half. Remove the chicken from the mixing bowl, drain it on kitchen paper and cut it into thin slices.

5. Chop the nuts roughly and mix well with the zucchini, chicken, mint, and lemon juice. Use salt and pepper to season and arrange in bowls.

Nutrition:

- Calories 399 kcal

- Protein 36 g

- Fat 26 g

- Carbohydrates 6 g

- Phosphorus 122.3 mg

- Potassium 0.29 mg

- Sodium 77.9 mg

26. Veal Kidneys

Preparation Time: 45 minutes

Cooking Time: 10 minutes

Servings: 4

Ingredients:

- 1 veal kidney 500 g

- Milk for inserting the kidney

- 1 onion 60 g, diced

- 1 clove of garlic, diced

- 2 tablespoons of olive oil

- 1 pinch of sugar 150 ml of dry sherry

- 50 g of whipped cream 1 fresh bay leaf

- Salt Pepper from the mill

- 1 tablespoon of finely chopped tarragon

Directions:

1. Cut the veal kidney in half lengthwise, separate it, rinse it well and cover it for about 45 minutes with milk, then remove it, dry it and cut it into bite-size pieces.

2. Heat-up oil in a pan, fry the kidney pieces quickly, remove them, and keep warm.

3. Sweat the onions plus garlic until translucent in the frying fat, sprinkle with the sugar, deglaze with sherry, put in the bay leaf, and cook for 5 minutes.

4. Season with salt and pepper, remove the bay leaf, and remove the sauce from the stove. Mix in the cream and half of the tarragon, add the juice and kidneys and warm them up carefully.

5. Arrange the kidneys in a preheated bowl and serve the remaining tarragon sprinkled with it.

Nutrition:

- Calories 99 kcal

- Protein 15.76 g

- Carbs 0.85 g

- Fats 3.12 g

- Sodium 178 mg

- Phosphorous 241 mg

- Potassium 272 mg

27. <u>Soy Lime Roasted Tofu</u>

Preparation Time: 15 minutes

Cooking Time: 1hour 35 minutes **Servings:** 4

Ingredients:

- 28 ounces of Extra-firm tofu, drained and cubed

Reduced:

- 2/3 cup of Sodium soy sauce

- 2/3 cup of Lime juice 6 tablespoons of Sesame oil, toasted

Directions:

1. In a bowl, mix oil, lime juice, and soy sauce. Toss in tofu. Refrigerate for 1 hour to marinate.

2. Set oven to 450 ° F.

3. Remove tofu from marinade and spread on 2 baking sheets with some spacing between the pieces. Roast for 20 minutes, as you turn halfway until golden brown.

Nutrition:

- Calories 163 kcal Fat 11 g Carbs 2 g

- Protein 19 g

28. Chicken Nuggets

Preparation Time: 5 minutes

Cooking Time: 20 minutes

Servings: 6

Ingredients:

- 2 cups of chicken, cooked

- 8 ounces of Cream Cheese

- 1 Egg

- ¼ cup of Almond Flour

- 1 teaspoon of Garlic Salt

Directions:

1. While the chicken is still warm, set it in an electric mixer and shred. In case you are using leftover chicken, warm it up for a short time.

2. Once the shredding is done, add all the remaining ingredients and mix it up.

3. Drop scoops of the mixture onto a greased baking sheet; flatten it into a nugget shape.

4. Bake it for 13 minutes at 350 degrees, until they turn golden and cooked.

5. Enjoy when hot!

Nutrition:

- Calories 150 kcal

- Fat 18 g

- Protein 15 g

- Carbs 1.8 g

29. Crab-Stuffed Avocado

Preparation Time: 10 minutes

Cooking Time: 5 minutes

Servings: 5

Ingredients:

- 1 pound of Crab

- 1 Avocado, ripe, pitted, peeled

- 2 tablespoons of Onion, finely chopped

- 2 tablespoons of Cilantro, chopped

- Salt

- Pepper

Directions:

1. Place the crab in the Instant Pot and add a cup of water.

2. Set the lid in place and the vent should point to "Sealing."

3. Set the IP to manual and cook for 5 minutes.

4. Quick-release pressure.

5. Take the crab out and let it cool.

6. Extract the meat from the crab and discard the shells.

7. In a bowl, combine the crabmeat and stir in the rest of the ingredients.

8. Refrigerate.

9. Serve chilled.

Nutrition:

- Calories 149 kcal

- Carbs 4.7 g

- Protein 13.2 g

- Fat 15.3 g

30. Thai Fish Curry

Preparation: 5 minutes **Cooking Time:** 10 minutes **Servings:** 6

Ingredients:

- 1/3 cup of Olive oil 1½ pounds of Salmon fillets

- 2 cups of Coconut milk, freshly squeezed

- 2 tablespoons of Curry powder

- ¼ cup of Cilantro chopped

Directions:

1. In your instant pot, add in all the ingredients. Apply a seasoning of pepper and salt. Give a good stir.

2. Set the lid in place and the vent to point to "Sealing."

3. Set the IP to "Manual" and cook for 10 minutes.

4. Quick-release the pressure.

Nutrition:

- Calories 470 kcal

- Carbs 5.6 g Protein 25.5 g

- Fat 39.8 g

31. Avocado Grapefruit Salad

Preparation Time: 5 minutes

Cooking Time: 20 minutes

Servings: 4

Ingredients:

- 2 Avocados, peeled, pitted and meat scooped

- 1 Grapefruit, red, peeled ¼ cup of Pomegranate seeds

- 1 tablespoon of Shallots, minced ¼ cup of Olive oil

- 1 tablespoon of Pomegranate juice Salt Pepper

Directions:

1. Squeeze some of the grapefruit to obtain the juice. Sprinkle over the avocados in a bowl. Spread over the remaining grapefruit and the pomegranate seeds.

2. In another bowl, mix olive oil, salt, pepper, pomegranate juice, and shallots. Sprinkle over the salad and enjoy.

Nutrition:

- Calories 335 kcal Fat 18 g Protein 3 g

- Carbs 28 g

32. <u>Protein-Free Bucatini with Broccoli</u>

Preparation Time: 15 minutes

Cooking Time: 10 minutes

Servings: 1-4

Ingredients:

- 300 g of Bucatini (or spaghetti) protein-free

- A pinch of salt

<u>For the dressing:</u>

- 400 g of broccoli 3 tablespoons of extra virgin olive oil

- 1 clove of garlic

- 4 anchovies in oil 10 g of pine nuts

- 2 tablespoons of grated Parmesan cheese

- 2 tablespoons of grated pecorino Romano (an Italian cheese)

- 1 chili

Directions:

1. Clean the broccoli by dividing the florets, wash them, and put them in a pot containing 4 liters of lightly boiling salted water. After 6-7 minutes, they will be cooked, so drain them.

2. Brown the garlic clove with the oil and anchovies in a large pan. When it is golden, remove the garlic and add the chili, pine nuts, and broccoli. Allow to flavor by stirring.

3. Separately, cook the Bucatini (or spaghetti) in 3 liters of slightly salted boiling water. Drain them al dente and cook them in the broccoli pan.

4. Finally, season them with the grated parmesan and pecorino. Serve immediately.

Nutrition:

- Calories 89 kcal

- Protein 4.54 g

- Carbs 8.1 g

- Fat 4.73 g

- Phosphorus 197 mg

- Potassium 680.4 mg

- Sodium 167.4 mg

33. Quinoa Porridge with Honeyed Almonds

Preparation: 5 minutes **Cooking Time:** 15 minutes **Servings:** 2

Ingredients:

Almonds:

- ½ cup of raw almonds, chopped

- 2 tablespoons of honey

Quinoa:

- 1 cup of dried quinoa

- 1¼ cups of milk or almond milk

- 1 cup of water 1 (2-inch) of cinnamon stick

- ¼ teaspoon of ground cardamom (optional)

- ¼ cup of dried cranberries 2 tablespoons of honey

Directions:

Almonds:

1. Preheat the oven to 350 °F. Line a sheet pan with parchment paper.

2. Stir the almonds and honey together in a mixing bowl until the almonds are coated.

3. Spread the almonds over the lined sheet pan and roast for 5 to 10 minutes.

4. Remove from the oven and allow to cool.

Quinoa:

5. While the almonds are in the oven, add the quinoa to a medium saucepan and pour in the milk and water.

6. Add the cinnamon stick and stir in the ground cardamom, if using, and dried cranberries.

7. Bring to a boil, then immediately reduce the heat to low and cover the saucepan. Cook for 15 minutes.

8. Remove from the heat, discard the cinnamon stick, and stir in the honey. Ladle into two bowls and top with the honeyed roasted almonds.

Substitution Tip: pre-prepared sliced, blanched almonds may be used in place of raw almonds without the need for chopping. You can also use ¼-teaspoon of ground cinnamon in place of the cinnamon stick.

Nutrition:

- Calories 720 kcal Total fat 23 g Total Carbs 113 g

- Fiber 10 g Sugar 50 g Protein 23 g

- Sodium 66 mg

CHAPTER 7. DINNER

34. Baked Garlic Ghee Chicken Breast

Preparation Time: 5 minutes

Cooking Time: 30 minutes

Servings: 1

Ingredients:

- 1 chicken breast

- 1 teaspoon of garlic powder

- 1 tablespoon of ghee

- 2 cloves garlic, chopped

- 1 teaspoon of sea salt

- 1 teaspoon of chives, diced

Directions:

1. Preheat oven to 350 °F.

2. Place the chicken breast on a piece of foil.

3. Season with sea salt, garlic powder, chopped fresh garlic.

4. Top with ghee and rub everything into the chicken breast.

5. Wrap the chicken breast in the foil and place it on a baking tray.

6. Bake for 30 minutes, or until chicken breast is cooked through, with a meat thermometer reading above 165°F.

7. Serve with more salt and ghee to taste. Cut the chicken breast into slices and sprinkle diced chives on top.

Nutrition:

- Calories 264 kcal

- Carbohydrates 6.1 g

- Fat 15.5 g

- Protein 23.7 g

35. Crispy Chicken Thighs

Preparation Time: 5 minutes

Cooking Time: 40 minutes

Servings: 4

Ingredients:

- 12 chicken thighs

- 4 tablespoons of Olive oil

- 2 tablespoons of Salt

- 2 sprigs fresh rosemary, chopped

Directions:

1. Preheat oven to 450° F. Rub salt on each chicken thigh and place on a greased baking tray. Drizzle the olive oil over the chicken thighs and top with the rosemary.

2. Bake for 40 minutes until golden and crispy. Enjoy!

Nutrition:

- Calories 713 kcal Carbohydrates 0 g

- Fat 56 g Protein 48 g

36. Chicken and Bacon Sausages

Preparation Time: 10 minutes

Cooking Time: 20 minutes

Servings: 12

Ingredients:

- 1 pound of chicken breasts

- 2 slices bacon, cooked, crumbled

- 1 egg, whisked

- 2 tablespoons of Italian seasoning

- 2 teaspoons of garlic powder

- 2 teaspoons of onion powder

- ½ teaspoon of salt

- ½ teaspoon of pepper

Directions:

1. Preheat the oven to 425 °F.

2. Put all the ingredients into a food processor and process well.

3. From the meat mixture form approximately 12 thin patties (½-inch thick) and place on a baking tray lined with foil.

4. Bake for 20 minutes, until a meat thermometer shows 170° F.

5. Serve immediately or store in the freezer for 4 weeks.

Nutrition:

- Calories 370 kcal

- Carbohydrates 3 g

- Fat 21 g

- Protein 40 g

37. <u>Bifteck Hache (French Hamburgers)</u>

Preparation Time: 15 minutes

Cooking Time: 20 minutes

Servings: 4

Ingredients:

<u>Burgers:</u>

- 1½ pound of ground beef

- 4 tablespoons of Ghee

- 1 onion, diced 1 egg

- 1 tablespoon of fresh thyme leaves

- ½ teaspoon of salt ½ teaspoon of pepper

<u>Sauce:</u>

- ½ cup of beef stock 2 tablespoons of Ghee

- ¼ cup of parsley, chopped

Directions:

<u>Burgers:</u>

1. Place 2 tablespoons of ghee into a frying pan and cook half the diced onions until translucent, about 2-3 minutes.

2. Allow the onions to cool and add them with the oil in the pan to a mixing bowl with the egg, ground beef, salt, pepper, and thyme leaves.

3. Mix well and form 8 patties.

4. In a frying pan, cook the hamburgers with 2 tablespoons of ghee until both sides are well browned, about 5-6 minutes per side.

Sauce:

5. Place the ghee into a frying pan and sauté the remaining half of the onions, until translucent, about 2-3 minutes.

6. Add the beef stock and let cook until reduced, about 2-3 minutes. Add in the parsley.

7. Serve the sauce with the burgers.

Nutrition:

- Calories 460 kcal

- Carbohydrates 1 g

- Fat 36 g

- Protein 35 g

38. <u>Lemon Ghee Roast Chicken</u>

Preparation Time: 10 minutes

Cooking Time: 1 hour 45 minutes

Servings: 8

Ingredients:

- 4 pounds of whole chicken, remove giblets

- 1 lemon, zested, sliced

- 1 lemon, halved

- ½ cup of ghee

- 1 tablespoon of salt

Directions:

1. Preheat the oven to 350 ° F.

2. Combine lemon zest and ½ tablespoon of salt and rub all over the chicken.

3. Sprinkle ½ tablespoon of salt into the chicken cavity and stuff with lemon halves and ¼ cup of ghee.

4. Brush the remaining ghee on the outside of the chicken.

5. Place the chicken in a roasting pan and arrange the lemon slices around the chicken.

6. Roast for 1 hour 45 minutes. Using a meat thermometer, cook until the internal temperature of the meat is 165 °F.

7. Let the chicken rest for about 10 minutes before slicing and serving.

Nutrition:

- Calories: 465 kcal

- Carbohydrates: 0 g

- Fat: 30 g

- Protein: 43 g

39.   Oven-Baked Parmesan Garlic Wings

Preparation Time: 5 minutes

Cooking Time: 30 minutes

Servings: 12

Ingredients:

- 6 pounds of whole chicken wings

- 8 tablespoons of butter, melted

- 1 egg

- ½ teaspoon of Italian seasoning

- ½ cup of Parmesan cheese

- 1 teaspoon of garlic powder

- ¼ teaspoon of crushed red pepper

- ¼ teaspoon of salt

Directions:

1. Preheat the oven to 425 °F and cut the wings into two pieces.

2. Put the wings on a baking sheet with a metal rack on top. Cook for 15 minutes.

3. Make the sauce by combining the cheese, butter, seasonings, and egg in a small bowl. Don't worry about using a raw egg in the sauce; the wings will be hot enough.

4. Remove the wings from the oven and flip them over. Turn on the broiler and broil for 5 minutes. Flip again and broil for another 5 minutes. Keep flipping and broiling until they are done to your desired crispness. They should reach an internal temperature of 165°F.

5. Toss immediately in the sauce.

6. Garnish with extra cheese.

Nutrition:

- Calories 602 kcal

- Carbohydrates 0.6 g

- Fat 45.9 g

- Protein 45.4 g

40. <u>Crispy Indian Chicken Drumsticks</u>

Preparation Time: 5 minutes

Cooking Time: 40 minutes **Servings:** 5

Ingredients:

- 2 pounds of chicken drumsticks 2 tablespoons of Salt

- 3 tablespoons of garam masala ½ tablespoon of coconut oil

Directions:

1. Preheat the oven to 450 °F.

2. Smear a large baking tray with coconut oil.

3. In a bowl, mix the garam masala and salt.

4. Pat the drumsticks dry.

5. Coat each drumstick with the mixture and lay it on the baking tray. Bake for 40 minutes. Serve immediately.

Nutrition:

- Calories 362 kcal

- Carbohydrates 3.6 g Fat 24.3 g

- Protein 34.7 g

CONCLUSION

Intermittent fasting is not a new direction of dieting. In fact, people have been doing it since the beginning of time. Certain fasts, such as the Ramadan fast, Lent, etc., have been practiced since ancient times. Though based on beliefs and religions, these fasts are still forms of intermittent fasts and have similar positive effects as well. Intermittent fasting basically means eating at particular times during the day and fasting for the remaining time. So, for instance, if you have your breakfast at 8:00 a.m., you are supposed to fast until 8:00 p.m. The fasting period allows your body a resting period and leads to weight loss, glucose regulation, and various other benefits.

There exist a variety of intermittent fasts. Some of them are easy to do, while some are quite difficult for beginners. Regardless of the ease of an intermittent fast, it can still be one of the most difficult things you ever do if you have never fasted before. You need to regulate your diet cycle, which can be quite a task for many. Yet, it can't be compared to the grueling fact that you need to go 'hungry' for 8-10-12 or even more hours of the day. Eating one or two meals per day and going 'hungry' for the rest is especially difficult for people with busy schedules who are often accustomed to eating anything they find whenever they get the time. Such people avoid doing intermittent fasting because they believe that they cannot stick to the diet or will go hungry.

CPSIA information can be obtained
at www.ICGtesting.com
Printed in the USA
LVHW081327220621
690776LV00010B/491

9 781803 008943